# A N G I N A

*learn about coronary heart disease*
*and how to prevent it*

by

## Julia Ann Purcell, RN, MN, FAAN

## Barbara Johnston Fletcher, RN, MN, FAAN

## Suzanne Cambre, RN, BSHA

This book is not meant to replace your doctor's advice or treatment. It is to help you understand the symptoms, treatment and prevention of coronary heart disease.

# WHY ANGINA?

Angina symptoms are your heart's way of telling you that it is not getting enough blood and oxygen. Most of the time angina is the result of fatty buildup in the coronary arteries that feed the heart. You may not feel any symptoms during the slow buildup. Then, one day, you may feel discomfort. If the symptoms are brief (5-10 minutes) and go away completely, they are called angina or angina pectoris. If the symptoms last longer than a few minutes, heart damage can occur (a heart attack). This does not have to happen!

There are things you can do to help your heart. As you read this book, you will learn how to respond to the symptoms of coronary heart disease (CHD). You will also find out how to change your life to prevent more fatty buildup in your heart's arteries. In the long run, you may be able to reduce fatty buildup or prevent cracks in the fatty plaque. Your actions will be the key to staying healthy and preventing heart damage.

# Table of Contents

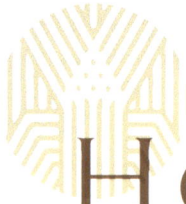

# How the Heart Gets Oxygen

The heart muscle gets oxygen from blood brought in by 3 major arteries and their smaller branches.

1. right coronary artery (RCA)

2. left anterior descending (LAD)

3. circumflex artery

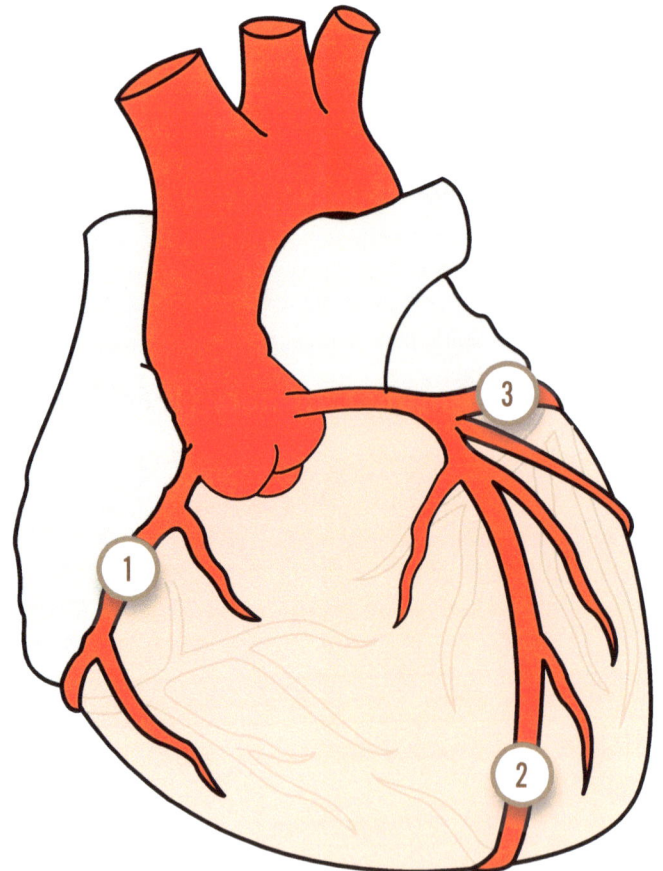

The heart has to have a steady supply of oxygen. Two problems in the coronary arteries that can keep the heart from getting enough blood and oxygen are:

- fatty deposits (atherosclerosis) that build up in the artery wall

- spasm (sudden squeezing of a coronary artery)

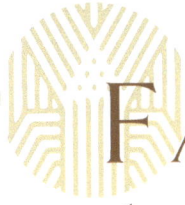

# FATTY BUILDUP (ATHEROSCLEROSIS)

High levels of cholesterol and blood fats can lead to fatty buildup in the arteries. There are 2 main types of cholesterol: High Density Lipoprotein (HDL or the "good" cholesterol) and Low Density Lipoprotein (LDL or the "bad" cholesterol). HDLs help get rid of the bad LDLs and lower total cholesterol. LDLs are attracted into the artery walls, causing fatty buildup. Triglycerides are another type of blood fat that plays a role in fatty buildup.

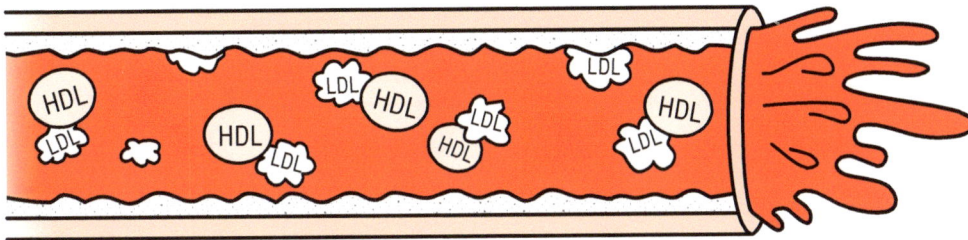

Fatty buildup is more likely when:

- your diet is high in **cholesterol and saturated fat**

- arteries have been **damaged by inflammation, high blood pressure** or **nicotine/tobacco**

- you **don't exercise**

- you are **overweight**

- you have **diabetes** or family history of coronary artery disease

- you are **tense** from too much stress

Most of the time, medicine is given to help reduce blood fat levels and reduce the risk of heart attack. Regular exercise, weight loss and a diet low in cholesterol and saturated fat will help lower LDL's and triglycerides and raise HDL's.

The fatty deposits (called **plaque**) build up slowly in the heart's arteries. When fatty buildup or a small clot narrows a coronary (heart) artery, less blood reaches the heart muscle. Angina symptoms occur when there is not enough blood and oxygen to meet the heart's needs. If angina symptoms last 5-10 minutes and go away completely, there is usually no heart damage.

## angina

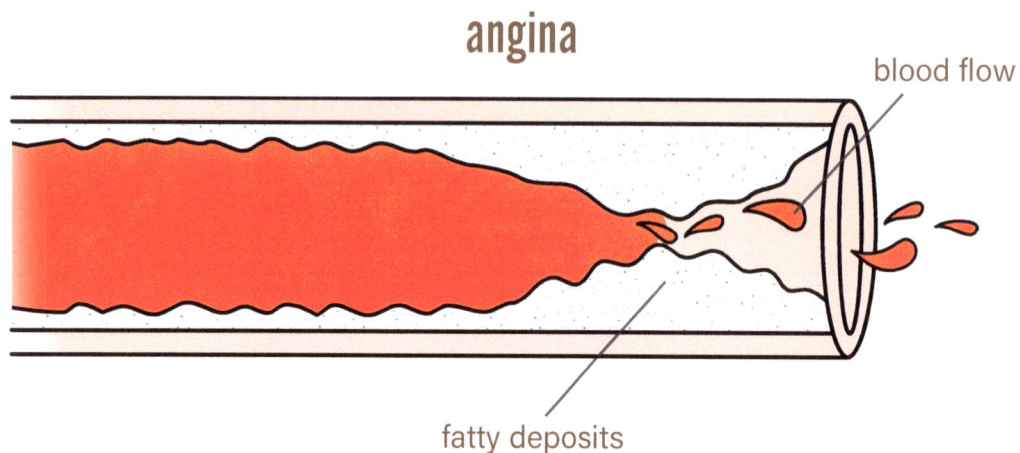

blood flow

fatty deposits

If a crack develops in even a small plaque, a blood clot may form. When a clot blocks the artery, no blood gets through. Heart damage (a heart attack) is likely, unless the artery can be opened within a few hours.

## heart attack

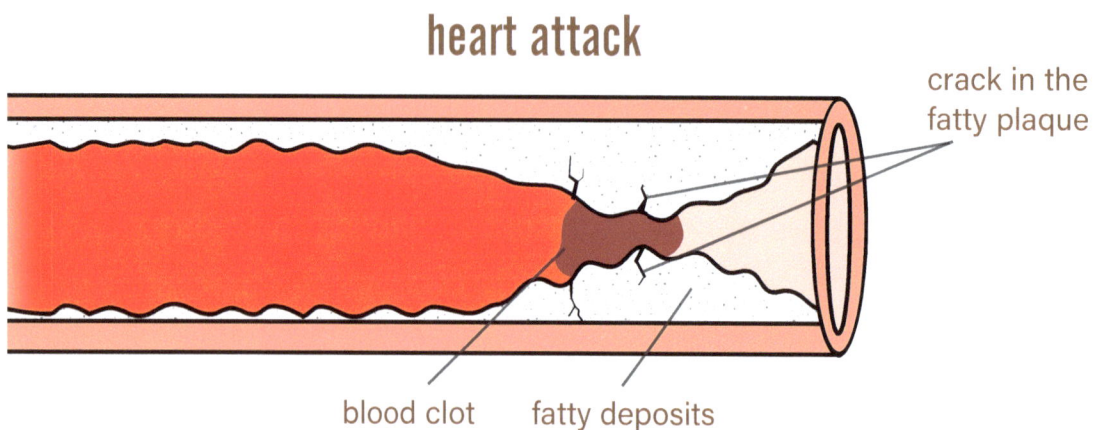

crack in the fatty plaque

blood clot     fatty deposits

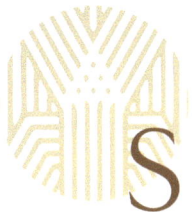

# SPASM

Spasm is not common in the coronary arteries. When spasm occurs, it DOES interfere with blood flow to the heart muscle. If the spasm is brief, it can cause angina symptoms. If spasm lasts longer than 10-15 minutes, heart muscle damage is likely (a heart attack). Both normal arteries and those with fatty buildup can go into spasm.

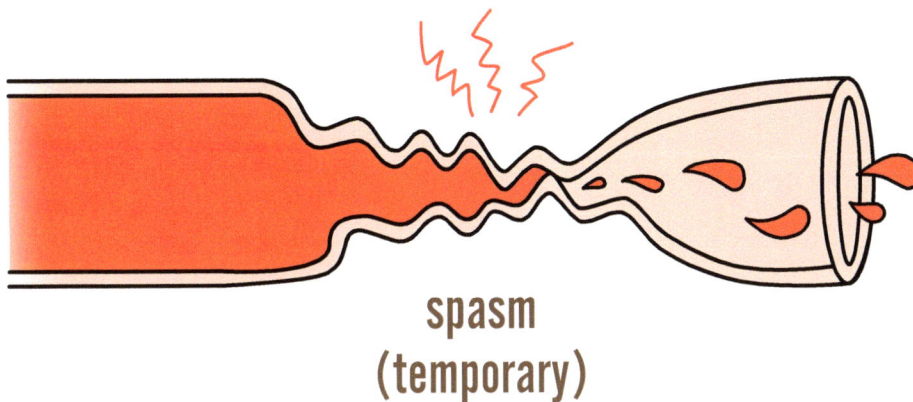

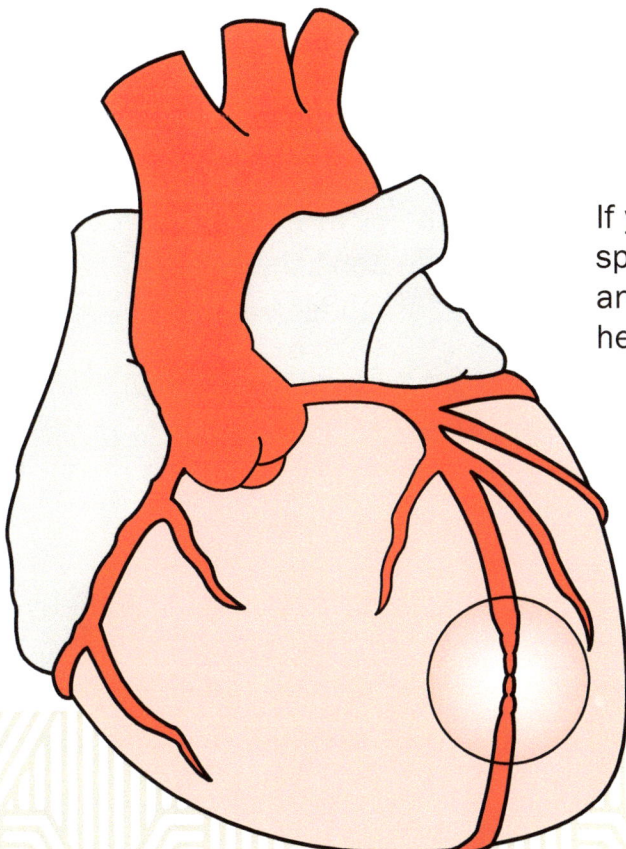

**spasm (temporary)**

If your doctor thinks coronary spasm is part of why you have angina, medicine to relax the heart arteries will be given.

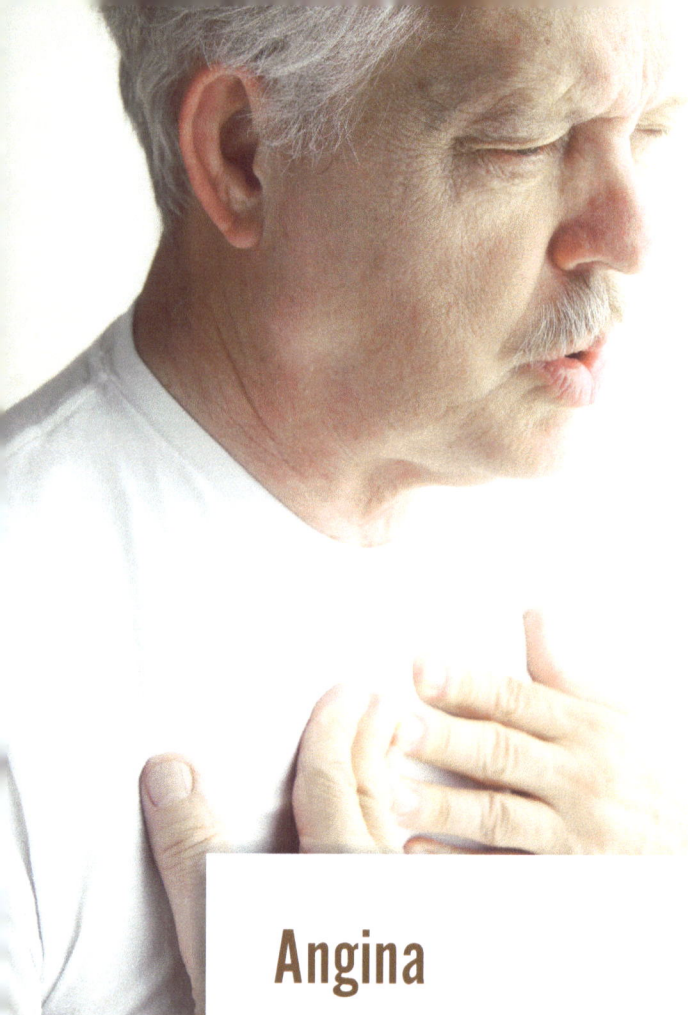

# Angina

When the heart needs more oxygen, most people have one or more of these symptoms:

- a tightening, pressure, squeezing or aching feeling in the chest or arms

- a "burning" feeling in the chest that may be confused with indigestion (heartburn)

- a sharp, burning or cramping pain or an ache that starts in or spreads to the neck, jaw, throat, shoulder, upper back or arms

Angina varies from mild discomfort in some people to pain in others. Some people feel breathless, weak or sweaty instead of any of the above.

Angina is more likely during physical work, mental stress, after heavy meals or in cold, windy weather. But you can have angina when you are resting. It may even wake you when you are asleep. Angina often goes away after you slow down or stop what you are doing. This can tempt you to ignore the feelings.

## Treat angina when you first feel it

NITROGLYCERIN (NTG) and REST are the quickest ways to relieve angina. Since angina is a warning that the heart needs more blood and oxygen, act fast when you **first** feel the symptoms.

Stop what you are doing and rest. Take a NTG tablet (or spray) under the tongue every 5 minutes (up to 3 tablets or sprays). **If you are not better in 15 minutes, call 911 or have someone drive you to the ER** (See more on page 10). **You need medical care NOW.**

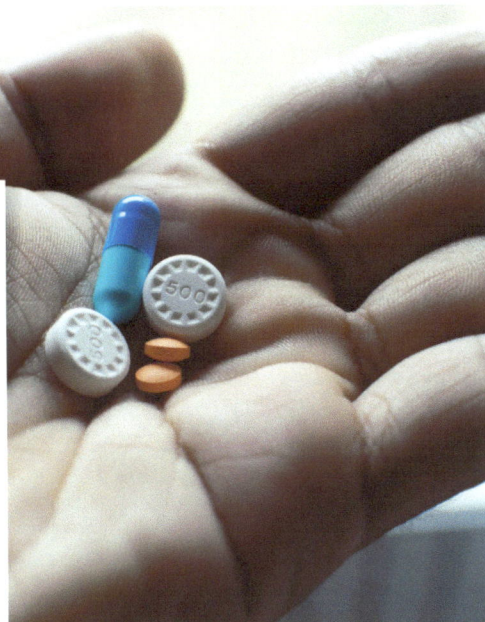

## More about NTG

A short-acting NTG tablet is a tiny white tablet which melts very fast when placed under the tongue. It does not work at all if swallowed. Keep the tablets in the brown bottle they come in. Keep tablets at room temperature. NTG tablets must be fresh in order to work. The tablets are usually fresh for one year after the bottle is opened. Replace them before the expiration date on the bottle.

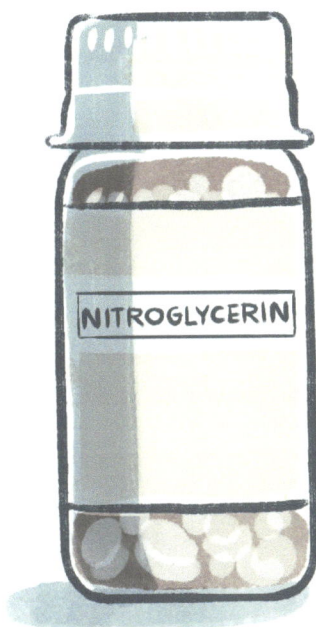

Short-acting NTG causes a brief headache for some people. If you take **either** an erectile dysfunction (ED) drug (Viagra®, Cialis®, or Levitra®) or a drug for lung high blood pressure (Revatio®, Adempas® or Adcirca®), DO NOT use any form of NTG for angina symptoms. See **A Word of Caution** on page 10.

## NTG Spray

NTG spray (Nitrolingual®) is a mist that should be sprayed onto or under your tongue. A full bottle of spray contains about 200 doses. The pump spray comes in a see-through bottle. Replace it when the fluid level is low. Bottles of NTG spray usually last about two years.

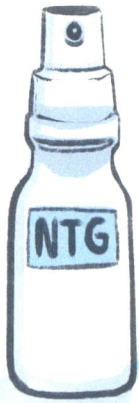

If angina is not relieved in 15 minutes by rest and NTG tablets (or sprays), call 911 or have someone take you to the nearest Emergency Room. If the pain is severe and you have other symptoms (shortness of breath, sweating, nausea, dizziness) don't wait 15 minutes to call 911. You may be having a heart attack. Have someone leave a message with your doctor's office.

Keep your short-acting NTG (tablets or spray) with you at all times. If a certain activity often causes angina, your doctor may tell you to take NTG beforehand. This may help prevent angina.

### A Word of Caution:

Erectile dysfunction (ED) drugs like Viagra®, Cialis® and Levitra® and drugs for lung high blood pressure (Revatio®, Adempas® or Adcirca®), can cause dangerous heart and blood pressure changes if taken within 24 hours of a short-acting or long-acting form of nitroglycerin. This includes amyl nitrate "poppers". If you have chest pain and have used one of these drugs in the past 24 hours, go straight to the nearest emergency room for help instead of taking NTG.

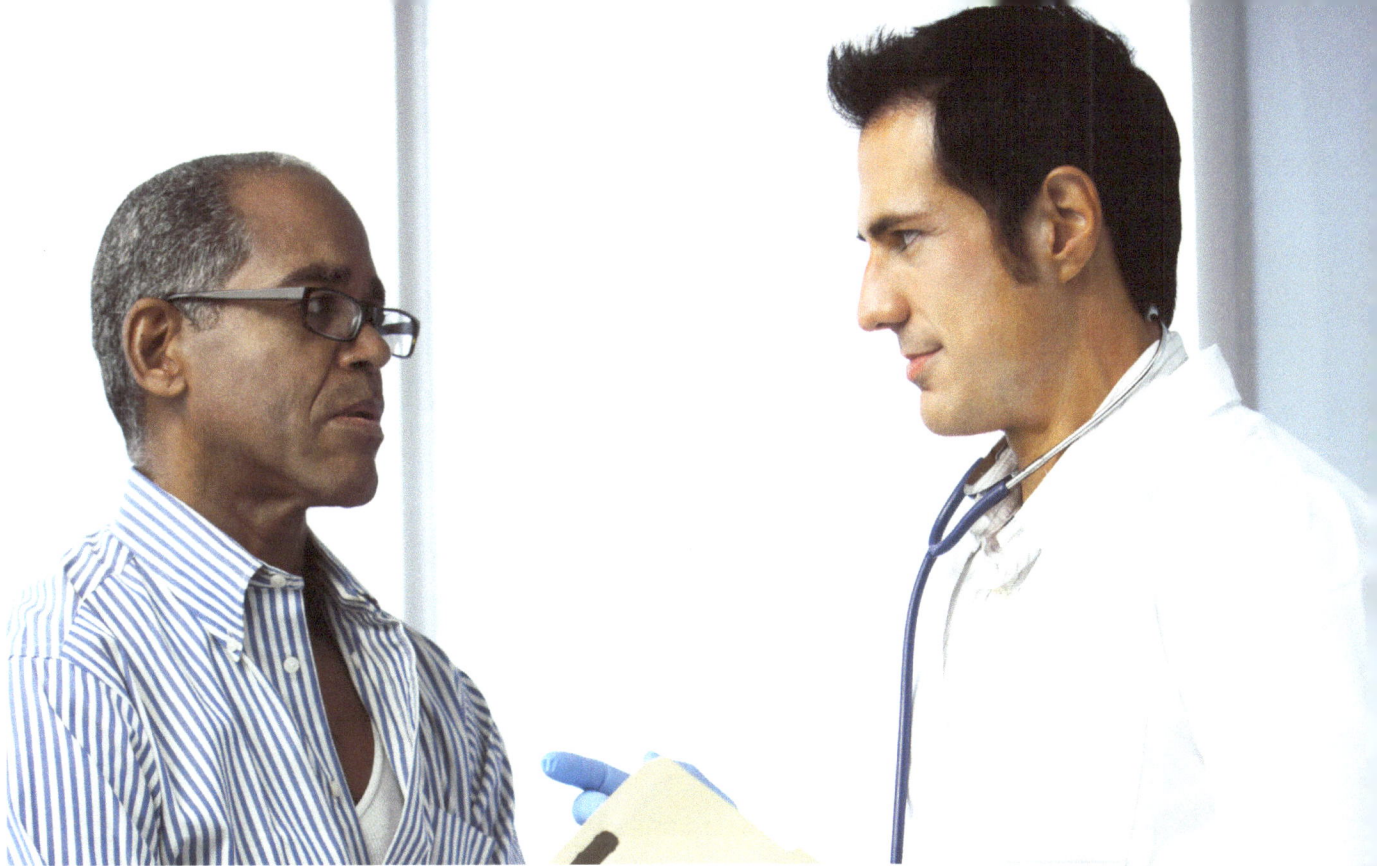

## What if your angina changes?

Be alert for any changes in your angina. Let your doctor know if your angina:

- comes on more often than usual or in a new area of the body

- occurs with less and less physical effort (or when you are resting)

- lasts longer each time

- takes more NTG than usual for relief

- wakes you in your sleep

Any of these can be a warning that the artery blockage is **more severe** with a greater risk of heart attack. Your doctor may use the term Acute Coronary Syndrome (ACS) to describe this change in angina.

If you have changes in your angina, see your doctor soon. Treatment may be needed to prevent a heart attack.

# Heart Attack

Suspect a heart attack and go to the emergency room if you feel pressure, tightness, heaviness, squeezing, burning or pain in the upper body that **lasts longer than 15 minutes.**\*  Just like angina, you can have these feelings anywhere in the upper body, including:

- the center of the chest

- the upper part of the stomach

- either arm

- the throat, neck or jaw

- the middle of the back or shoulder blades

15 minutes

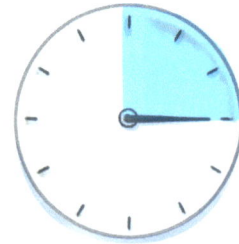

The discomfort can stay in one part of the body or move into the back, either arm or the neck.

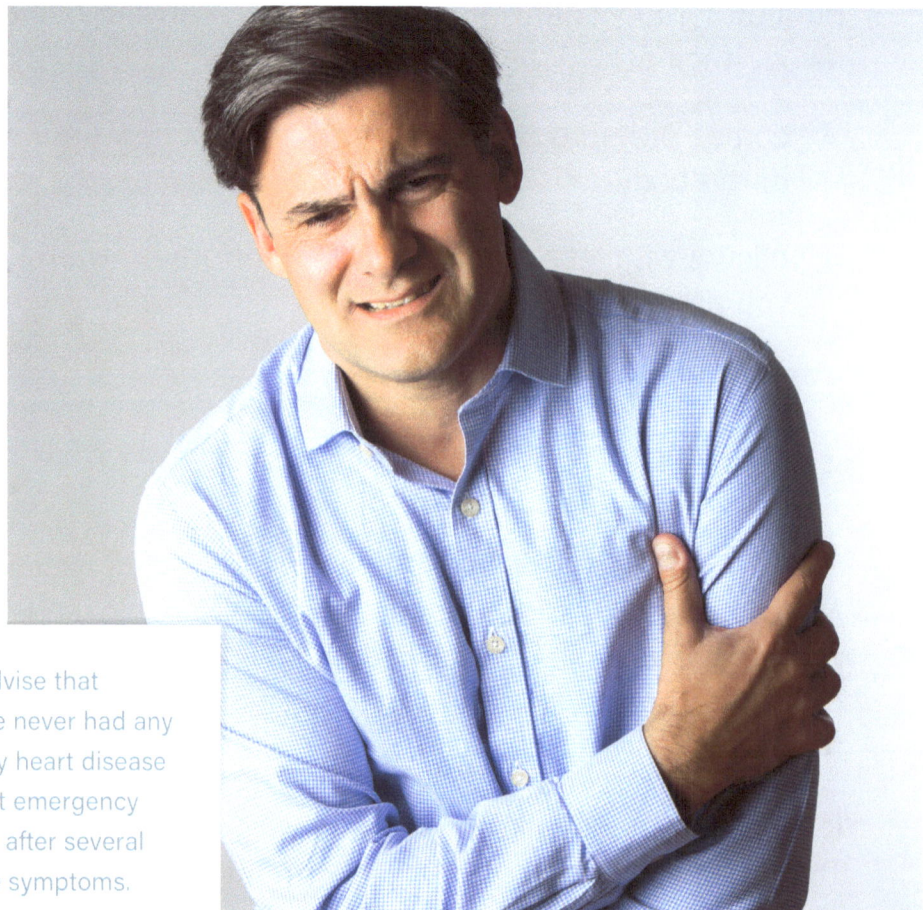

\*Some experts advise that people who have never had any signs of coronary heart disease go to the nearest emergency room right away after several minutes of these symptoms.

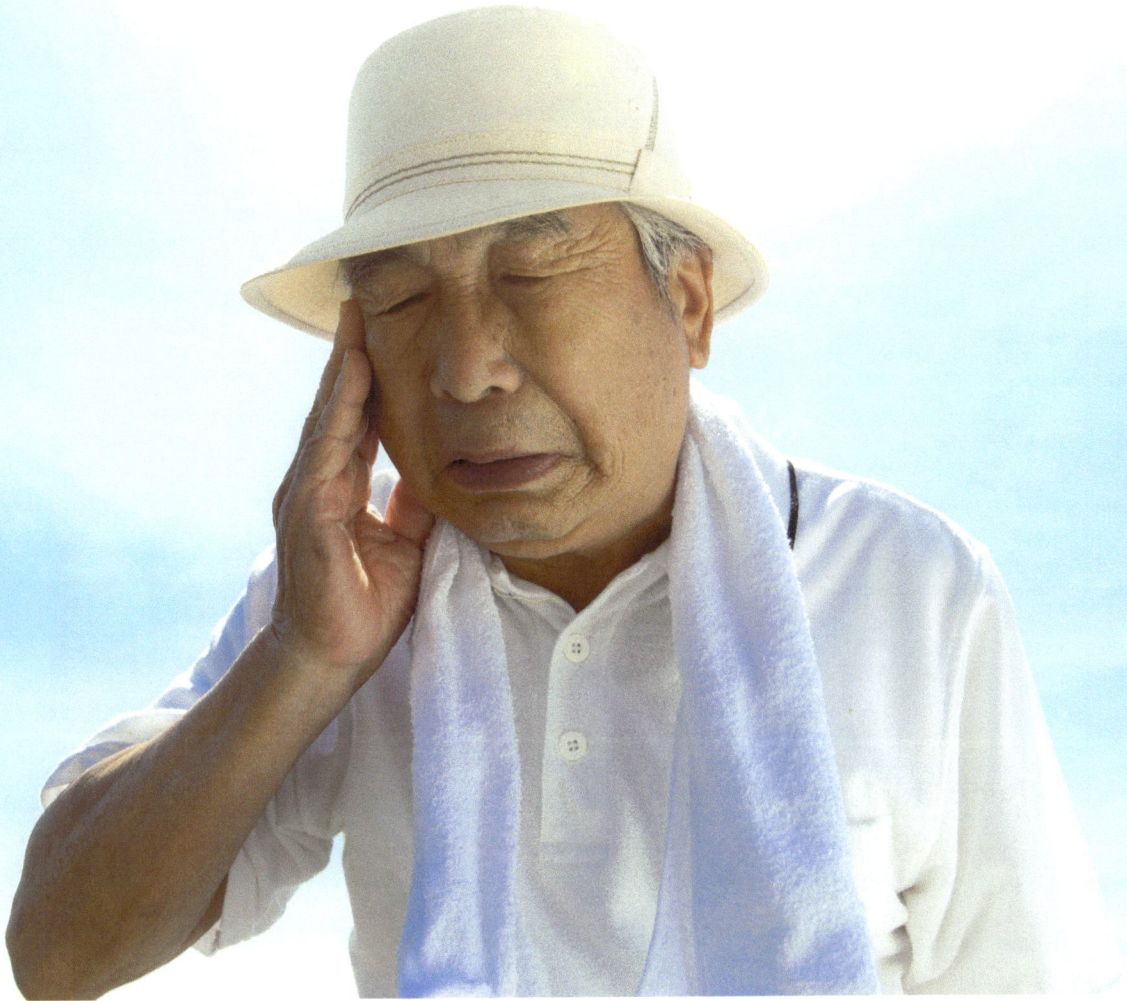

The pain of a heart attack is not always severe. Sometimes other symptoms go along with a heart attack such as:

- sweating

- nausea and vomiting

- shortness of breath

- feeling weak, faint or dizzy

- heart palpitations or skipped heartbeats

The symptoms of a heart attack may get worse or better, but you should always let your doctor know right away if you are having them.

Women often take longer to recognize their heart attack symptoms and delay seeking help. Many report that their heart attack symptoms were less intense than they had imagined and often included shortness of breath, nausea, fatigue and/or dizziness.

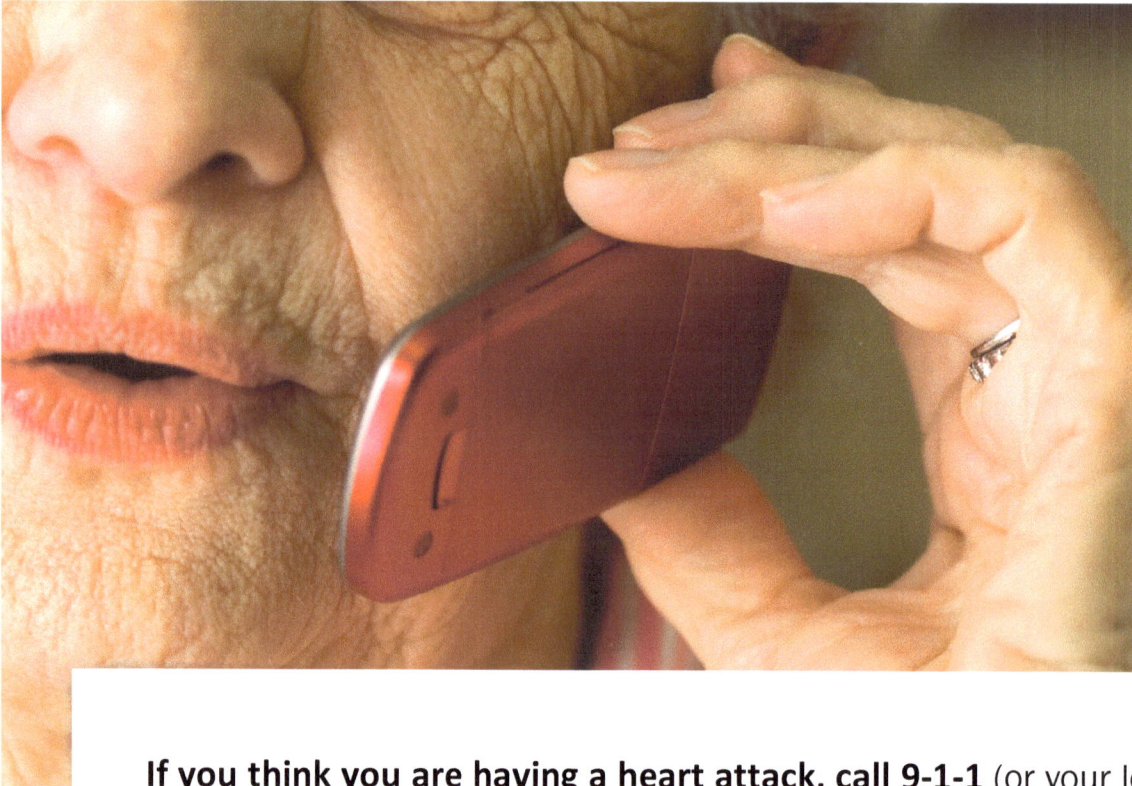

**If you think you are having a heart attack, call 9-1-1** (or your local rescue service number*)!  Minutes do matter!  Emergency Medical Technicians (EMT's) can start life-saving care and in many cases, alert the hospital before your arrival.  While you wait, chew a non-coated aspirin unless you have an allergy to aspirin.  If you are alone, unlock your door, and sit or lie down.  Loosen any tight clothes and take slow deep breaths.  Call and ask someone to come sit with you.

A heart cath (catheterization) is often done right away to see if blood flow can be improved with a balloon procedure (angioplasty[†]). Sometimes a drug can be given to dissolve a blood clot in a blocked artery.  These drugs are called "clot busters" (thrombolytics).  If blood flow can be restored quickly, less heart damage is likely.

People with very little heart damage can go home in a few days.  Others have more damage and may take longer to recover.  The size of a heart attack can be limited by fast action.

*If you are in an area without 9-1-1, do as the local emergency rescue personnel advise to get the quickest help for a heart attack. DO NOT drive yourself.

[†]See page 30 for more information about angioplasty and stents.

# Preventing Angina

Have regular medical checkups and get an annual flu shot. Take your meds as you are told and make some heart-healthy changes in your life.

## Long-acting NTG

Long-acting forms of nitroglycerin come in:

- **tablets or pills**

- **skin patches**

- **ointment**

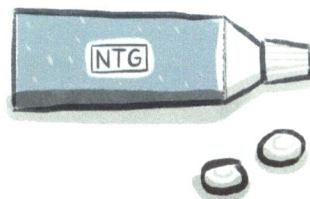

The skin patch and ointment have the longest effect of any kind of NTG. When using one of these, do this:

- Use a different site on your upper arm or upper body (front or back) each time you put on a patch. The patch works best if you avoid skin with hair, rash, cuts, scars or callouses. Keep the patch away from skin folds like under the breast or at the bend of your inner arm.

same time
every day

- Remove the old skin patch and put on the new patch at the same time each day. Don't cut it. After a bath, wait until your skin is dry to put on the patch.

- If the patch gets wet while you swim or bathe, it's OK. Water will not keep it from working.

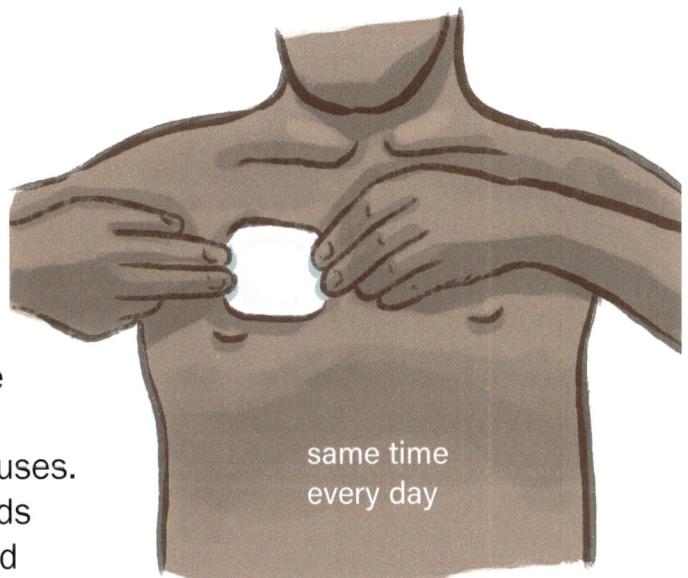

*Note:*

See *A Word of Caution* on page 10 about not taking any form of NTG if you have used an erectile dysfunction drug or a drug for lung high blood pressure within the last 24 hours.

## Other medicines

Most people with narrow heart arteries take a drug(s) to help keep blood cholesterol and fats in normal range. A 'statin' (Lipitor® or Crestor®) is often used but others include a resin, fibrate, cholesterol-absorbing drug (Zetia®) or niacin. Omega-3 fatty acids from fish or fish oil capsules may also help. New drugs that lower LDL are available for some.  These drugs require that you (or someone else) give yourself a shot (Repatha® or Praluent®).

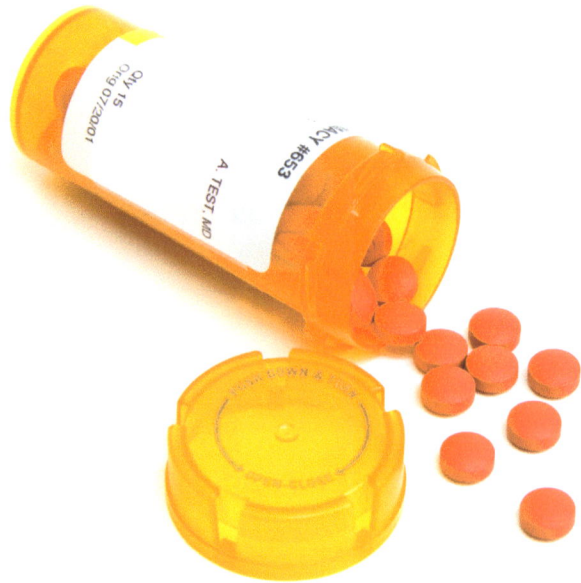

In addition, a drug(s) from these groups is often used for persons with coronary heart disease:

- Beta-blockers
- ACE inhibitors (or ARBs)
- Calcium channel blocker
- Late sodium-channel blockers

A **beta-blocker** helps the heart beat slower and use less oxygen during hard physical activity or mental stress.  It can also lower high blood pressure but doesn't often affect normal blood pressure.

A **calcium channel blocker** is used to prevent artery spasm. It also helps relax arteries all over the body making it easier for the heart to pump.  It also often helps lower high blood pressure.

An **ACE inhibitor** (or ARB) may help prevent or lessen the changes in heart size and shape that can occur with coronary heart disease.  It also relaxes body arteries to reduce the work of the heart.  MDs often prescribe one of these when angina occurs along with high blood pressure, diabetes or kidney disease.

A **late sodium channel blocker** drug like **Ranexa**® allows the heart to relax a bit more between heartbeats.  This gives time for the heart arteries to relax between heartbeats, and more time for coronary artery blood flow.   Ranexa® does not affect your heart rate or blood pressure so it can be used with other angina medications.

**Anti-platelet drugs** like aspirin and/or Plavix®, Effient®, or Brilinta® help prevent blood platelets from 'clumping' together to start a blood clot. **If your doctor asks you to take a daily aspirin by itself or along with another anti-clotting drug, be sure you know the correct dosage.** Often only a small dose (81 mg) is needed. Never take a daily dose of aspirin on your own! Sometimes, an anticoagulant ("blood-thinner") like Coumadin®, Pradaxa®, Eliquis® or Xarelto® is used instead of an anti-platelet drug. When Coumadin® is used, frequent blood tests and dose changes are needed. Be sure to tell any doctor you see about your anti-clotting drug(s) including any aspirin if ordered.

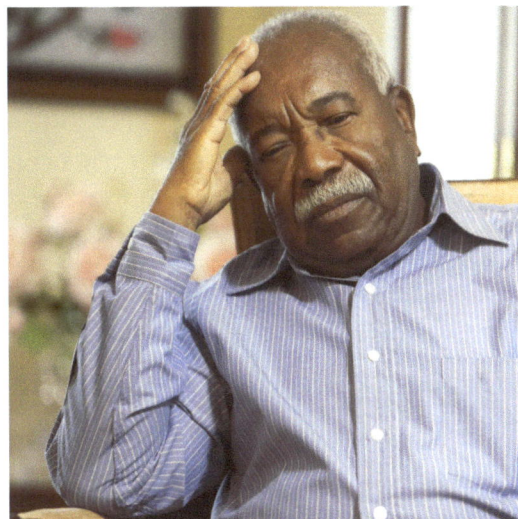

Since **bleeding** can occur with an anti-platelet drug or a 'blood thinner', call your doctor if you have severe bruising, prolonged nose bleeds or severe unusual headache, or other signs of bleeding.

Any of the drugs used for angina can cause milder side effects. Let your doctor know if you become light-headed, have swollen ankles or a dry cough, or notice a change in:

- energy
- bowel habits
- mental state
- sex drive or performance
- breathing
- appetite or food tolerance

You may need a different dosage or kind of medicine.

This chart is for a list of your medicines and how to take them. You may want to make a copy of the list to carry with you in your wallet or purse.

| Name | How much / how often | Time of day | | |
|------|----------------------|-------------|---|---|
| | | | | |
| | | | | |
| | | | | |

## Make some changes

The pace of your life has a lot to do with how often you have angina. The heart needs more oxygen when you are in a hurry, very active or upset. Slowing down can reduce the heart's need for oxygen.

Rest after meals. Give your heart a chance to pump blood to the stomach where food is being absorbed. Avoid mental stress and heavy exercise just after eating. Eat a number of small meals instead of 1 or 2 large meals each day.

Cut down on things that seem to cause your angina or make it last longer than usual. Limit walking up steep hills and a lot of steps. Limit hard work like raking leaves, lifting heavy things and straining to open windows or tight jar lids.

If you notice angina about the same time each day, find ways to make it easier for your heart. Take a short rest or slow your pace at that time.

rest after meals

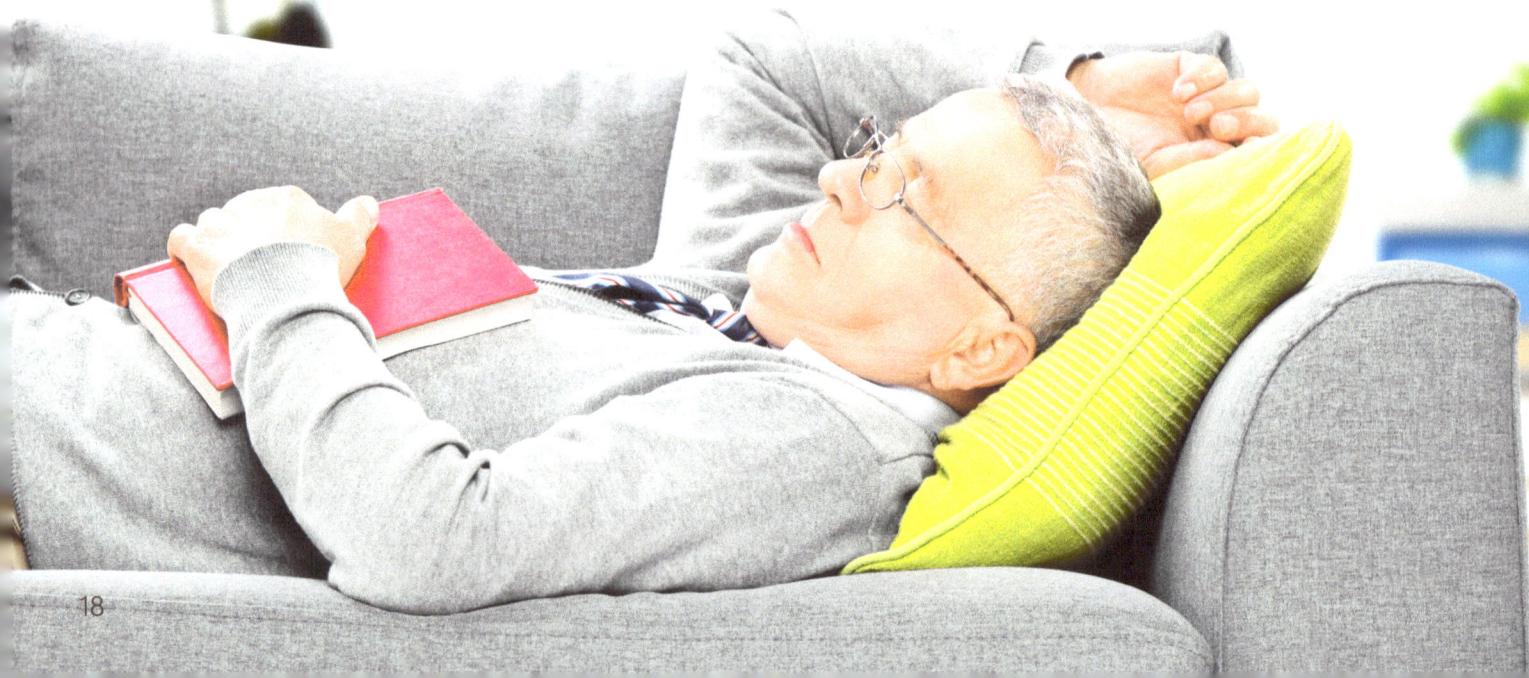

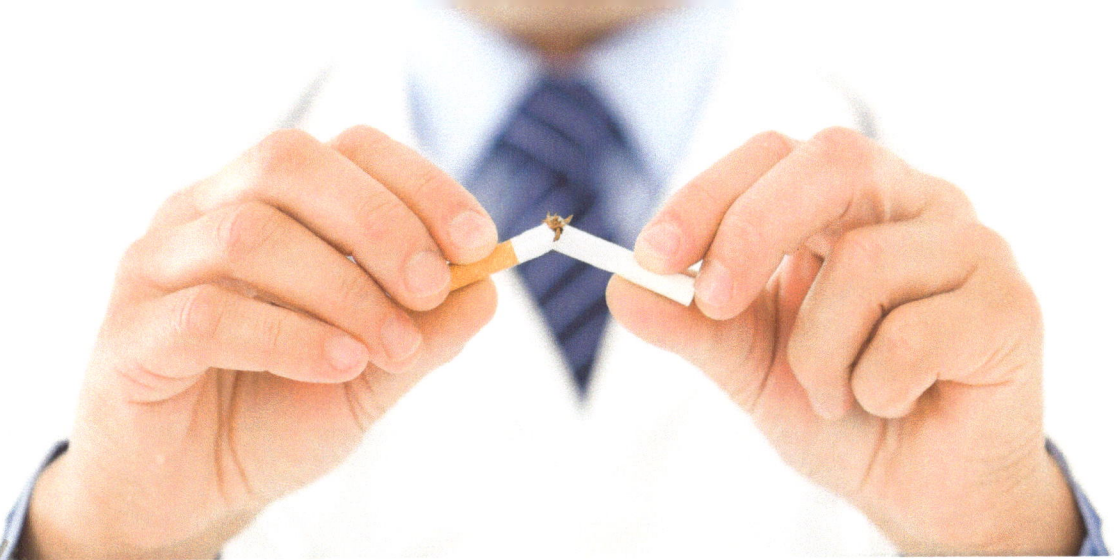

# PREVENTING CORONARY HEART DISEASE

Changes in your **risk factors for coronary heart disease** can not only prevent fatty buildup in the body arteries, but also may help get rid of blockage already there.  The goal for you is to make changes in your lifestyle to slow or stop the fatty buildup in your arteries.

## Smoking

Smoking is one of the worst things you can do to your body.  Breathing others' smoke is also harmful.  Snuff, chewing tobacco and nicotine contained in 'e' cigarettes also increase your risk of coronary heart disease.  Nicotine damages the lining of your arteries and tightens them so less blood and oxygen get to the heart.  Smokers who have coronary heart disease are at greater risk for heart attacks and sudden death.  If you stop smoking, these risks start to subside within 90 days.  Nicotine-replacements (gum, lozenges, patches, sprays or inhalers) help some people stop smoking.  Others become non-smokers by taking a prescription drug like Chantix® (varenicline) or Wellbutrin®.  These drugs block the flow of brain chemicals that make you want to smoke.

# High blood pressure

High blood pressure is often the result of tightening of arteries in the body. High blood pressure causes wear on the artery linings. This makes it easier for fat in the blood to move into the artery walls. Over time, the fat becomes hard. This keeps the arteries from relaxing enough for a lower pressure.

The pre-treatment goal for your blood pressure at rest should be less than 140 (top number) and less than 90 (bottom number). Studies continue to look at whether an ideal resting BP should be less than 120/80 for most patients. Your doctor will set a BP goal for you as goals vary with age and other medical conditions. To control high blood pressure and limit artery damage:

- eat a balanced, low-saturated fat, low-sodium diet (aim for 1500 mg/day of sodium and less than 10% of calories in saturated fat)

- lose weight (if you are overweight)

- take the prescribed medicine(s)

- exercise

- don't smoke and avoid secondhand smoke at work, home, or public places

- limit alcohol to 1 drink a day (women) or 2 drinks a day (men)

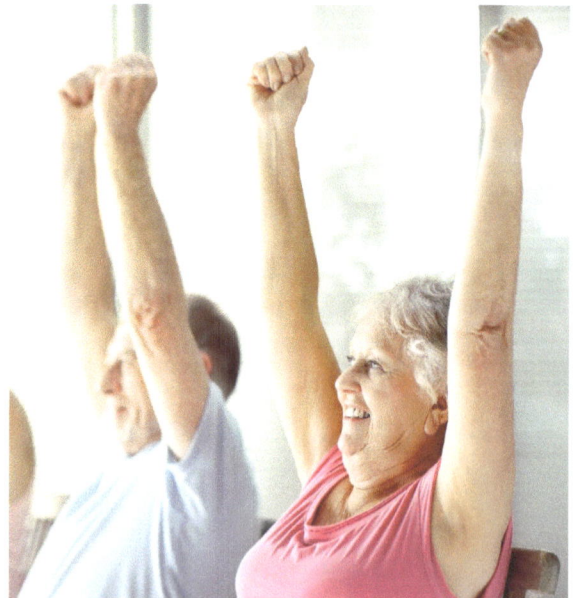

With exercise and weight loss, many people can reduce high blood pressure to the point they no longer need blood pressure medicine.

**1 drink =**

- 1.5 oz 80 proof liquor **or**

- 4 oz wine **or**

- 12 oz beer

# High blood fats

A **diet high in fat and cholesterol** adds to the blood fat made by your body. The more fat in your blood stream, the easier it is for some of it to move into the artery wall. Keep your saturated fat intake less than 5-6% of your daily calories. Goals to lower blood fats are:

- **total cholesterol** = less than 200 mg/dL

- **LDLs** (the 'bad' cholesterol) = less than 100 mg/dL*

- **HDLs** (the 'good' cholesterol) = more than 40 mg/dL (men) and 50 md/dL (women)

- **triglycerides** = less than 150 mg/dL

- **Non-HDL cholesterol** (total minus HDLs) = less than 130 mg/dL*

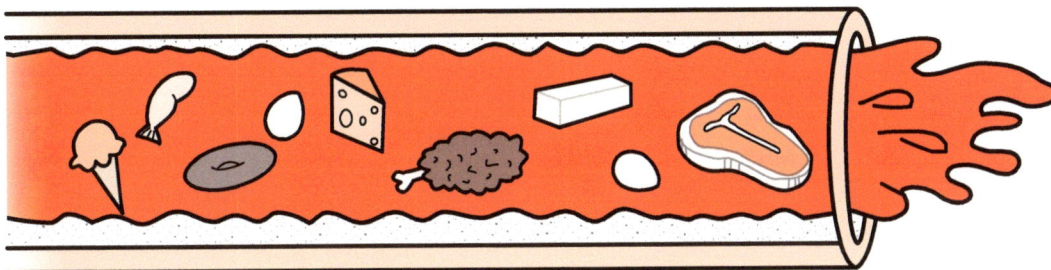

*If you are at high risk of heart attack, your goals may be an LDL less than 70 mg/dL and a non-HDL cholesterol of less than 100 mg/dL.

**Most people need a drug to lower cholesterol, LDLs and triglycerides and raise the good cholesterol (HDLs).** A heart-healthy diet, more physical activity and weight loss (if needed) can be very helpful. Studies show you may be able to reduce fasting triglycerides down to 100 mg/dL. Heart-healthy eating means more fruits, vegetables, whole grain foods and high-fiber foods and no more than 6 oz/day of lean meat, poultry (no skin) or fish. Avoid processed foods and sugar-added beverages/foods. Aim for 1500 mg/sodium intake per day.

The American Heart Association suggests the heart-healthy **DASH** diet (Dietary Approaches to Stop Hypertension) and aiming to eat less than 1500 mg sodium/day. You can find out about it online at www.dashdiet.org or in a bookstore (example: *The DASH Diet Action Plan* by Marla Heller). **Read food labels with care and avoid all foods with trans fats!** Trans fats are found in high-fat baked goods, hard margarines and foods with partially hydrogenated vegetable oils. Avoid pre-packaged/ processed foods and fast foods. Keep your saturated fat intake less than 5-6% of your daily calories. Choose low-fat dairy dairy products (milk, cheese, frozen desserts). Limit red meat as well as foods and drinks that are high in sugar and salt. Use less fat in your cooking, and when you do, use one of these:

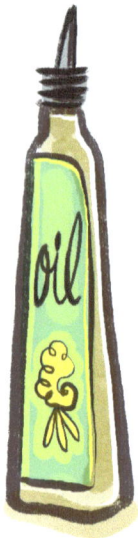

- monounsaturated oil (canola, olive, peanut)

- polyunsaturated oil (safflower, sunflower, corn, soybean, sesame)

Here are some low-fat ways to cook your food: **bake, broil, poach, grill, steam** or **stir fry** (with very little oil). Trim all fat off meat before cooking. It's OK to cook poultry with the skin on, but don't eat the skin as a lot of fat sticks to it. Season foods with herbs, low-sodium spices, fruits and vegetables.

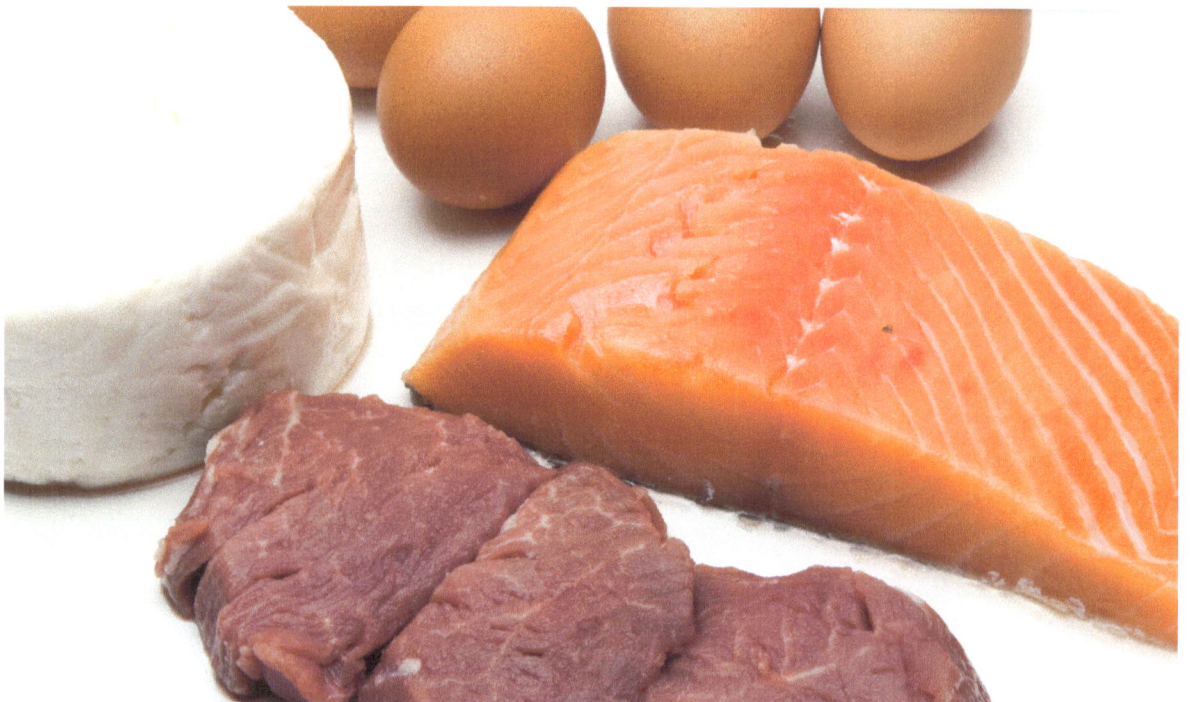

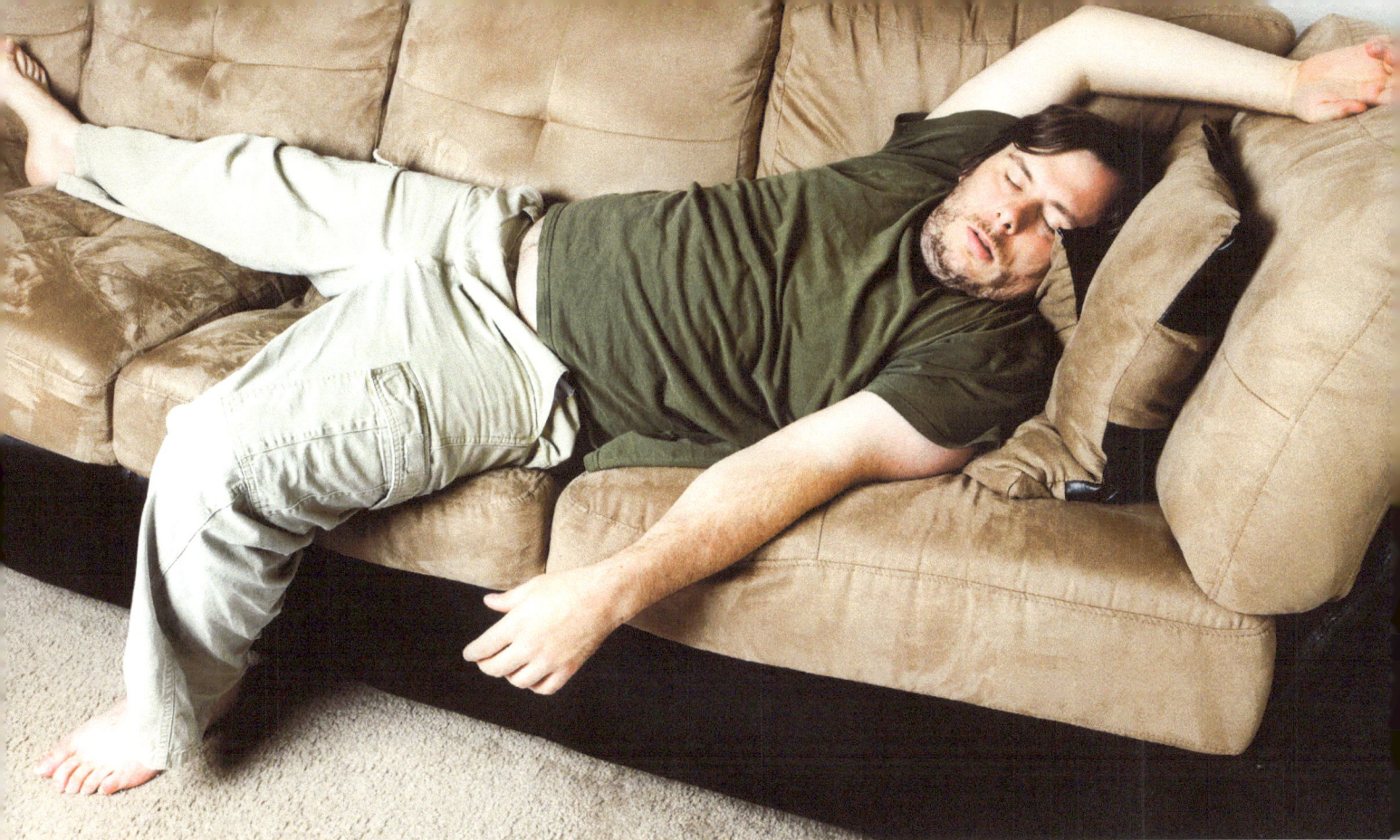

## Lack of exercise

Consider a regular exercise program: 30-60 minutes a day, 5-7 days a week. Exercise can raise the body's good cholesterol and better control fatty buildup in the arteries. Exercise and diet can help you lose weight, feel more relaxed and lower blood pressure and blood sugar.

If you exercise 30-60 minutes/day at least 5 days a week, the heart should be able to do more work with less effort. If you have angina, you may not be able to play sports like singles tennis, basketball or football. Things like golf, doubles tennis, walking, fishing, short swims and sex are OK for most people with angina.

Since your heart needs more oxygen during exercise, always check with your doctor before starting any exercise program. Pick an exercise you like that matches what your heart can do. A cardiac rehab program can help you with an exercise plan suited just for you. It can also help you in changing your other risk factors.

# Overweight

People who are overweight increase their risk of heart disease. You can tell if you are overweight by your:

- BMI (Body Mass Index)

- "waist" size (measured at top of hip bones)

tape measure

hip bone

leg

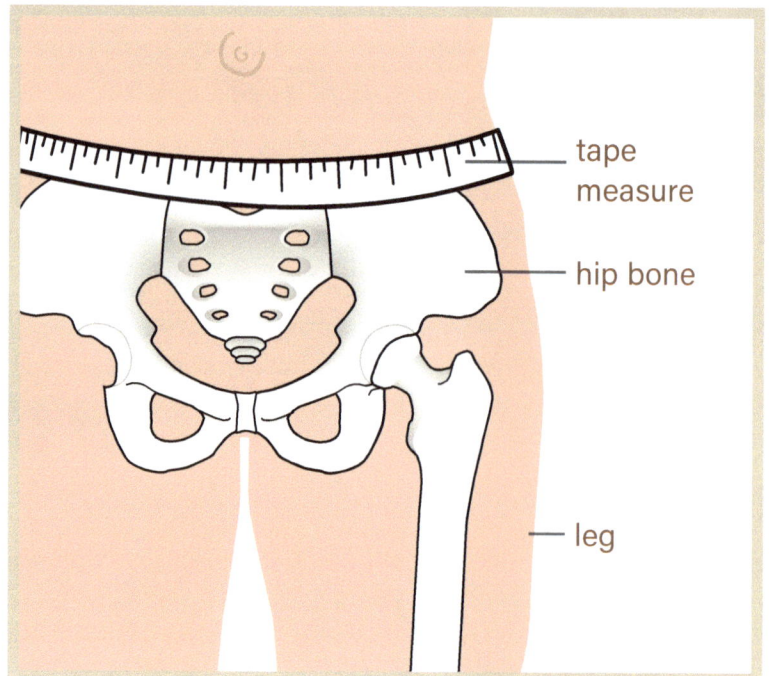

If your body mass index is less than 25, you are in a healthy weight range. If your BMI is between **25-29.9**, you are **overweight** and **30 or higher**, you are considered obese. Ask your doctor for your BMI or you can figure it for yourself at http://www.bmicalculator.org.

Your "waist" size also tells if you are overweight. Female waist size should be less than 35 inches and males less than 40 inches. The way you "wear" your weight is also a factor. Apple-shaped people (weight around the middle) are more likely to have heart disease than pear-shaped people (weight around the hips).

Choose a diet that lets you lose weight slowly. The DASH diet comes in these options: 1200, 1600 or 2000 calorie options/day. Ask your doctor or dietitian to help you. Don't choose diets that claim fast weight loss in a short time. Very low-calorie diets (under 1000 calories/day) can be dangerous. Anyone on such a diet should be under a doctor's care.

## Stress and tension

Emotional stress is any pressure from the outside that makes us feel tense on the inside. Stress comes at us from all sides, and can lead to depression if we don't handle it well. Since stress makes the heart work harder, try to find ways to relieve the pressure when you feel stressed. Many people find yoga, meditation and regular, suitable exercise helpful.

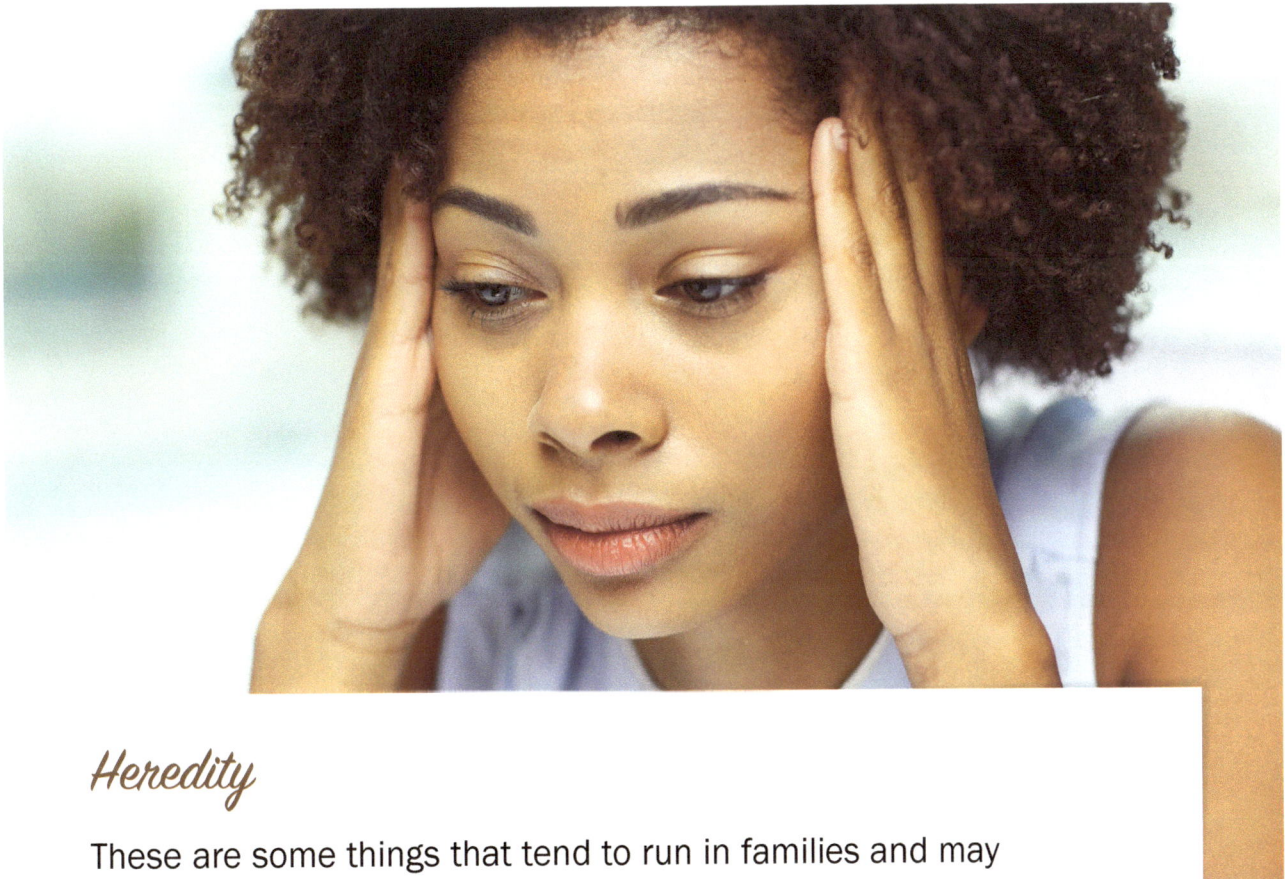

## Heredity

These are some things that tend to run in families and may lead to heart disease:

- high blood fat levels

- high blood pressure

- angina or heart attack at a young age
  (less than 55)

- diabetes

If heart disease runs in your family, it is even more important that you get rid of or control any other risk factors.

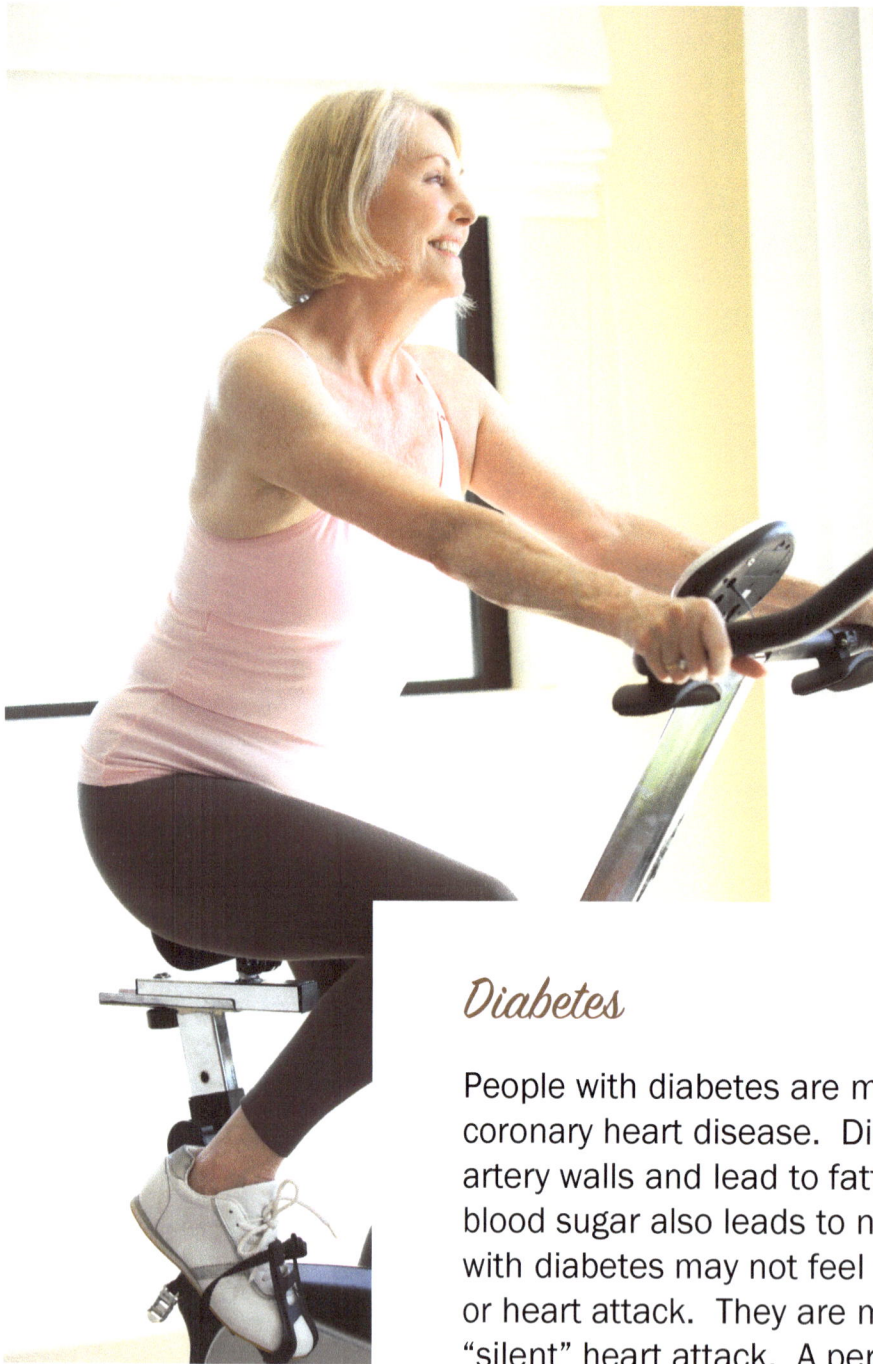

## Diabetes

People with diabetes are more likely to have coronary heart disease. Diabetes can damage artery walls and lead to fatty buildup. Since high blood sugar also leads to nerve damage, people with diabetes may not feel symptoms of angina or heart attack. They are more likely to have a "silent" heart attack. A person with diabetes must be alert to **any** symptoms of angina or a heart attack and take fast action. Proper diet and exercise may help lower your blood sugar. Fasting blood sugars should be less than 100 mg/dL and A1C* less than 6.5%.

*A1C is a special hemoglobin only produced by your body when blood sugar is high.

# *Make the changes that apply to you*

Making lifestyle changes will not only help prevent fatty buildup in the future but will make less work for your heart right now. Make your plans to:

- stop smoking

- lower high blood pressure

- eat a diet low in sodium (1500 mg/day), saturated and trans fats as well as cholesterol

- exercise regularly

- keep an ideal weight

- control stress and tension

- control high blood sugar (fasting sugars less than 100 mg/dL and A1C less than 6.5%)

With lifestyle changes and taking your medicines as prescribed, you may have less angina.

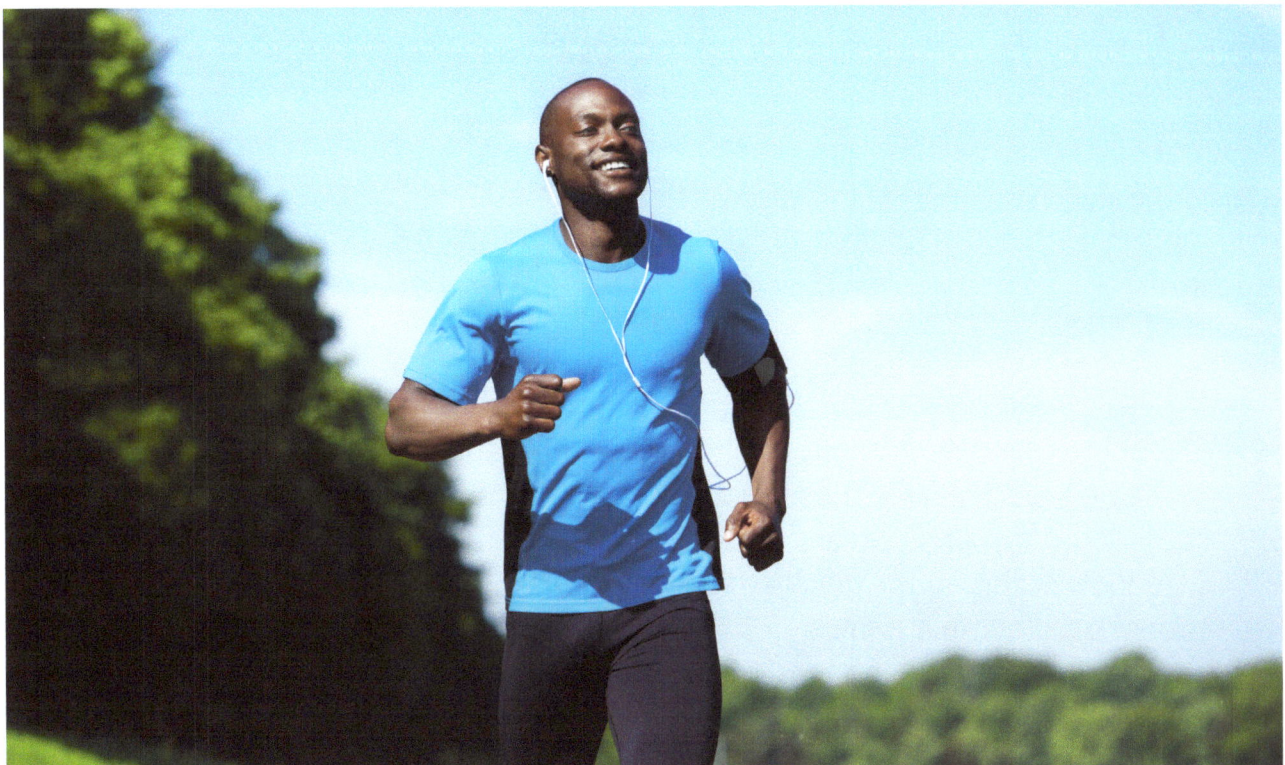

# TESTS

These are some of the tests that may be done to find out if there is blockage in the heart arteries and whether the symptoms are likely to lead to a heart attack in the near future.

**Resting EKG's** record the electrical activity of the heart and may show changes before, during or after a heart attack. EKG changes often occur during times when the heart needs more oxygen.

An **exercise test** can be useful if your doctor thinks you have blockage in a heart artery. An EKG and blood pressures are taken while you walk on a moving belt (treadmill) or ride a bike.

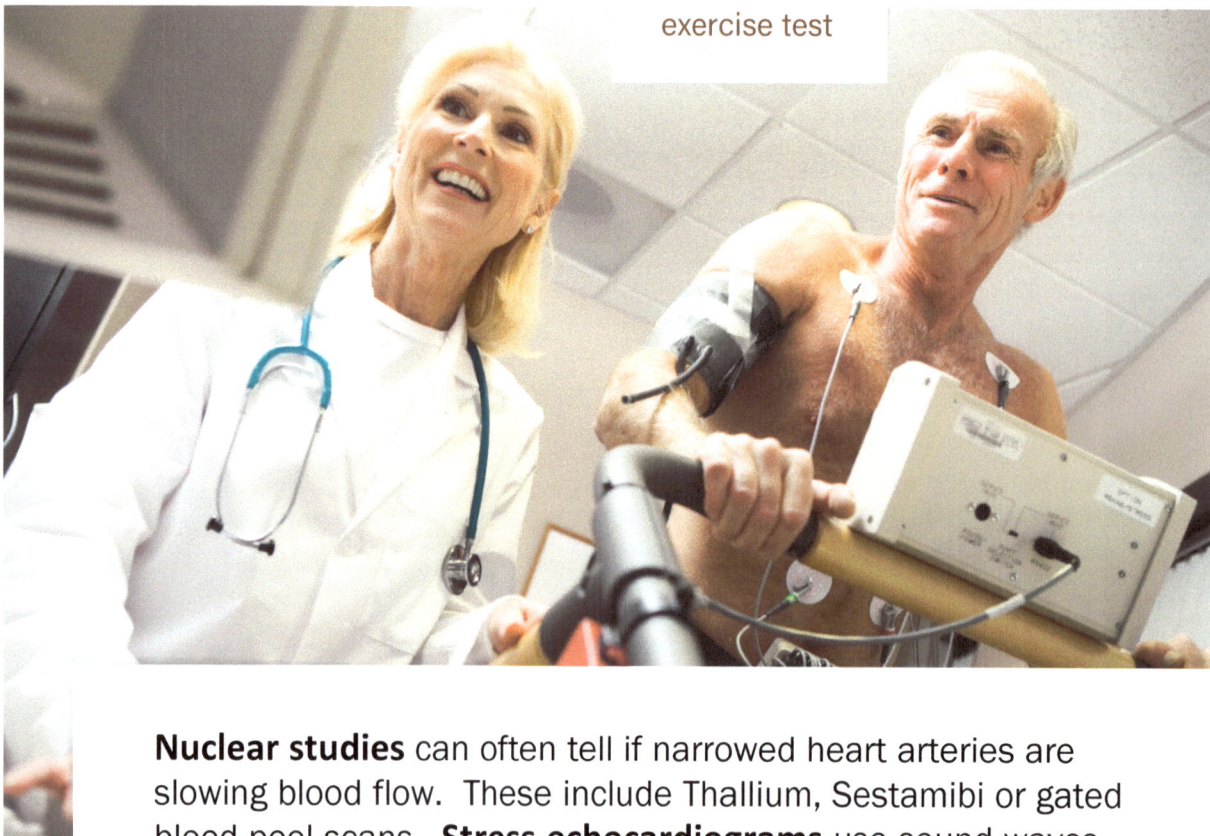

exercise test

**Nuclear studies** can often tell if narrowed heart arteries are slowing blood flow. These include Thallium, Sestamibi or gated blood pool scans. **Stress echocardiograms** use sound waves to look at the heart muscle. Both nuclear studies and stress echocardiograms can be done with an exercise test or by giving medicine to make the heart pump harder and faster.

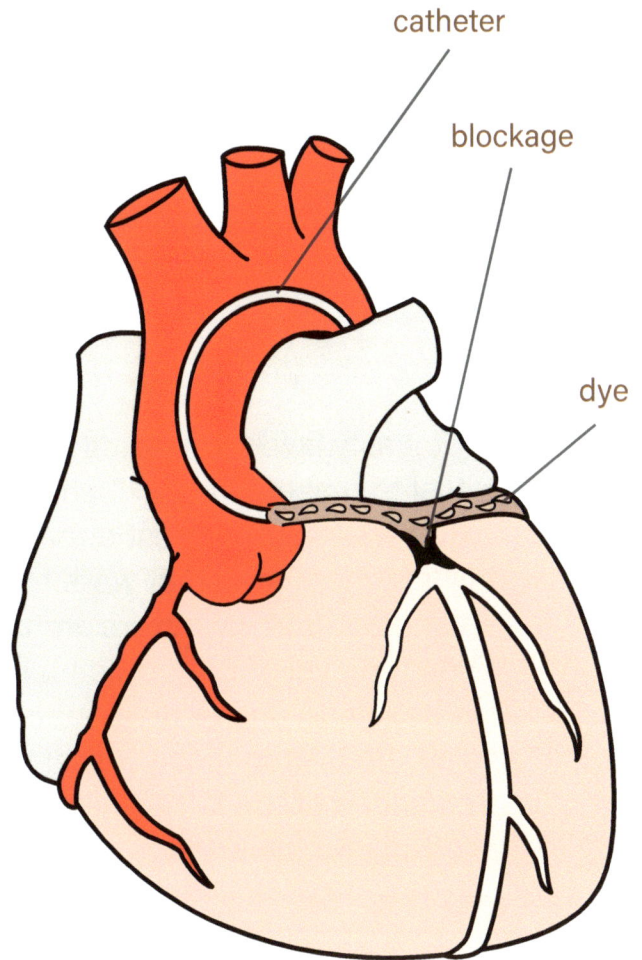

catheter

blockage

dye

**Cardiac Tomography (CT)** scans use x-ray to take painless heart pictures. During cardiac CT, the x-ray camera moves around the chest and the computer combines the images in a 3D view of the heart. Since an x-ray camera is used, some radiation is involved. Doctors in many hospitals are finding ways to do a cardiac CT with less radiation than before. In some cases, contrast ("dye") is given in a vein during cardiac CT to get more detail about the heart arteries. An **Ultrafast CT** is a less expensive cardiac CT looking for calcium in the heart arteries.

**Magnetic Resonance Imaging and/or Angiography (MRI or MRA)** of the heart give images of all parts of the heart including the heart arteries. The MRI scanner makes a magnetic field and transmits a signal to the heart. Pictures then come from the heart back to the scanner and the doctor looks for blockages. There is no radiation with an MRI.

Many times a **heart catheterization** (angiogram or dye test) is needed to see details of blockage in the heart arteries. A small catheter (tube) is guided into a blood vessel in your leg or arm and passed up to the heart. Once the catheter is in place, "dye" is injected and x-ray moving pictures are made of the heart's coronary arteries. This test also shows the pumping strength of the heart muscle and how well the valves are working.

# Treatments

Medicine, rest and changes in lifestyle can relieve or prevent angina. But if tests show that artery blockage is about to cause heart damage, angioplasty or bypass surgery may be needed.

## Angioplasty and Stents

Angioplasty involves placing a catheter (tube) in a narrowed blood vessel to make a bigger channel for blood flow. Although **balloon catheters** are used most often to inflate and compress the fatty buildup, there are other ways to widen a narrowed artery. Sometimes **cutting balloon catheters** are used to make tiny cuts in the fatty layers. When removal of fatty build-up is needed, an **atherectomy** catheter can be used. One or more stainless steel coils (stents) are often left inside the dilated blood vessel to help keep it open. If close-up pictures are needed of the fatty blockage, a special ultrasound catheter can be inserted into the artery.

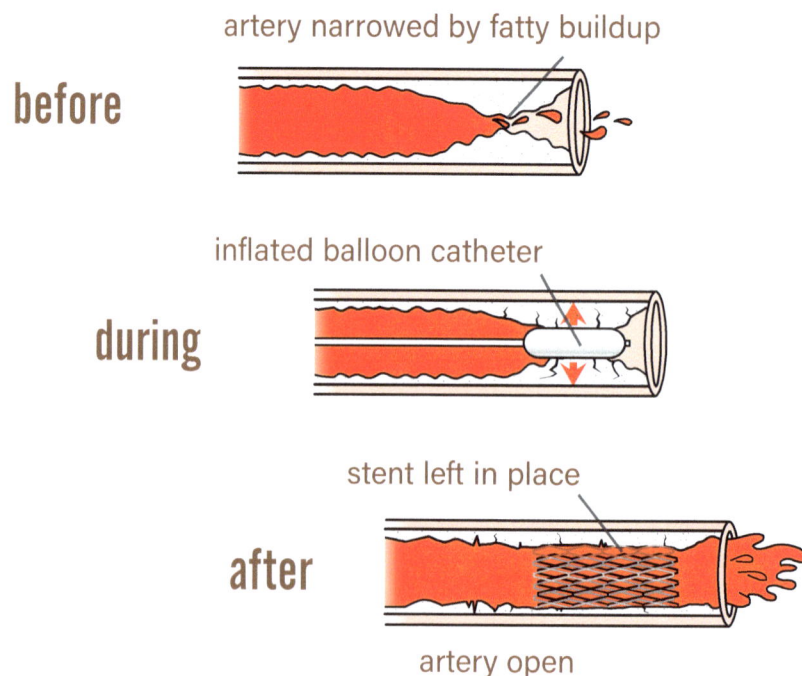

artery narrowed by fatty buildup

**before**

inflated balloon catheter

**during**

stent left in place

**after**

artery open

Rapid growth of smooth muscle cells at the angioplasty site can block heart arteries widened by angioplasty. This is called **restenosis.** Sometimes radiation (called **brachytherapy**) is used inside a stent to get rid of or block smooth muscle cell growth (in-stent restenosis). Most of today's stents are coated with a drug to slow buildup of smooth muscle cells (restenosis) after angioplasty. Studies continue with stents that are either partially or fully absorbed over time. However, stents can't be placed in all narrowed arteries.

## Bypass surgery

This surgery is sometimes needed to bypass several blockages in the coronary arteries and increase blood flow to the heart muscle. A leg vein or an artery from the chest is used for the bypass graft.

Recovery is longer for bypass surgery than for angioplasty.  But it may be the treatment of choice when a number of blockages are present. If angioplasty doesn't work, bypass surgery can be life-saving.

Your doctor will advise you about the treatment choices for your coronary artery blockage.

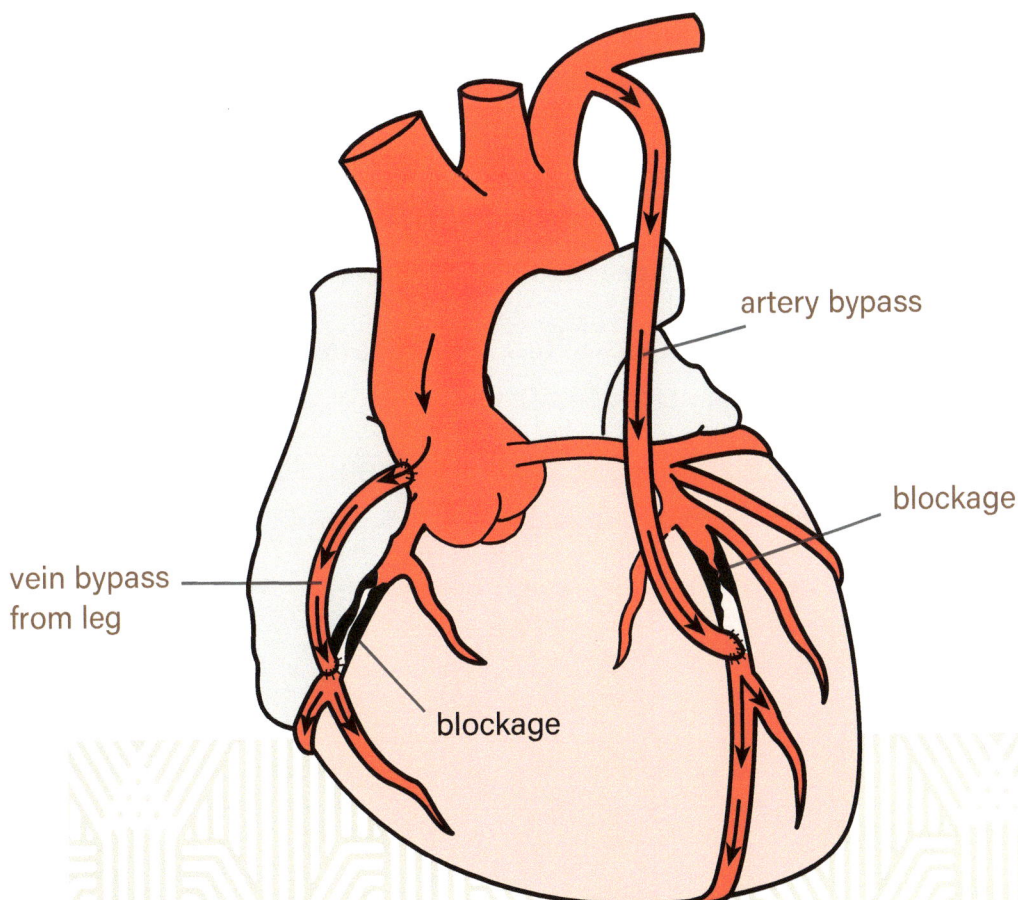

artery bypass

blockage

vein bypass
from leg

blockage

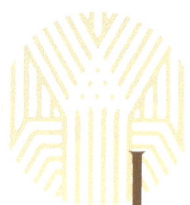

# LOOKING AHEAD

As research tells us more about the causes of coronary heart disease, we are better armed to control or prevent it. New tests are found and current treatments are improved nearly every week, including:

- gene testing/altering to:

  - correct high blood pressure, abnormal cholesterol levels and diabetes

  - determine antiplatelet drug dosage for prevention of blood clots **and/or**

  - to detect coronary artery disease (peripheral gene expression)

- techniques to encourage growth of new blood vessels in the heart (angiogenesis)

- improved drug-coated stents to help keep arteries opened with angioplasty from closing up again

- blood tests that detect inflammation in the heart arteries and warn of a heart attack

- improved exercise programs for people with limited blood supply to the heart

- better medicines for the heart and blood vessels and better use of medicines already available

- new findings about alternative therapies to help prevent coronary artery disease

Controlling risk factors is the key to preventing coronary heart disease. We hope this book will help you make choices for a healthier lifestyle.

# QUESTIONS TO ASK

Make a list of questions to ask your doctor or nurse about how to live well with angina. You may want to ask about:

- becoming a non-smoker

_____

_____

- blood cholesterol and fat goals

_____

_____

- daily calories for DASH diet and, if needed, weight loss goals

_____

_____

- a safe 30-60 minute, 5-7 days/week exercise routine

_____

_____

- blood pressure goals

_____

_____

- scheduling regular checkups and annual flu shot

_____

_____

www.ingramcontent.com/pod-product-compliance
Lightning Source LLC
Chambersburg PA
CBHW060854270326
41934CB00002B/129